Getting a Blood Test

A TODDLER PREP™ BOOK

About Toddler Prep™ Books

The best way to prepare a child for any new experience is to help them understand what to expect beforehand, according to experts. And while cute illustrations and fictional dialogue might be entertaining, little ones need a more realistic representation to fully understand and prepare for new experiences.

With Toddler Prep™ Books, a series by ReadySetPrep™, you can help your child make a clear connection between expectation and reality for all of life's exciting new firsts. Born from firsthand experience and based on research from leading developmental psychologists, the series was created by Amy Kathleen Pittman — mom of two who knows (all too well) the value of preparation for toddlers.

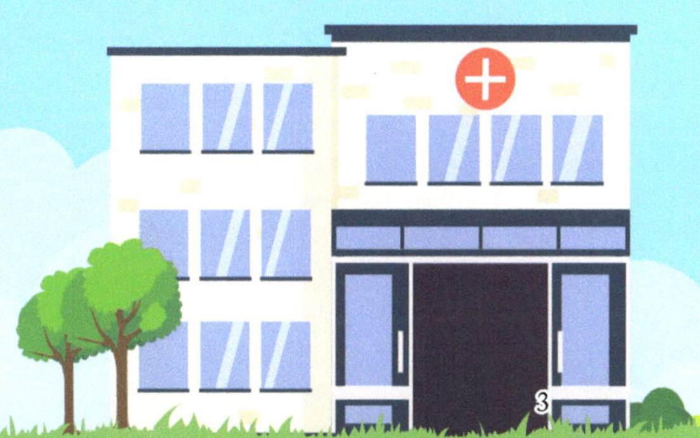

We're going to get a blood test. This helps us learn about your body. Let's talk about what happens when you get a blood test.

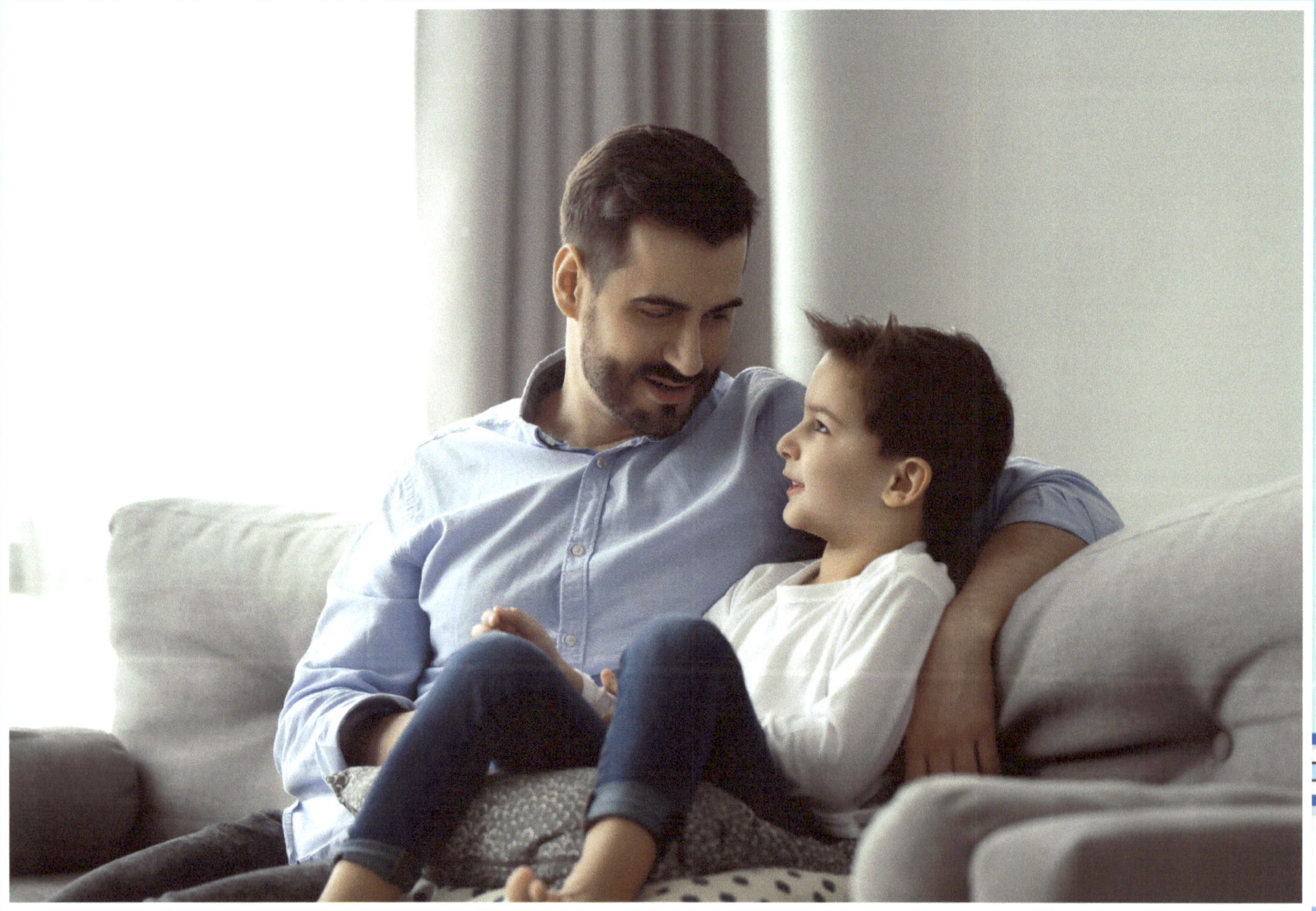

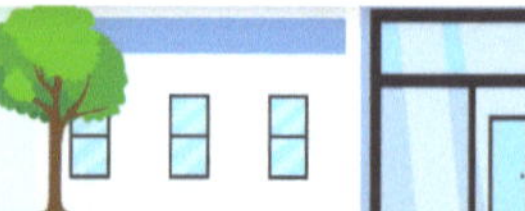

Blood is the red fluid inside your body. It carries food, air, and other things your body needs. It also helps fight germs when you are sick.

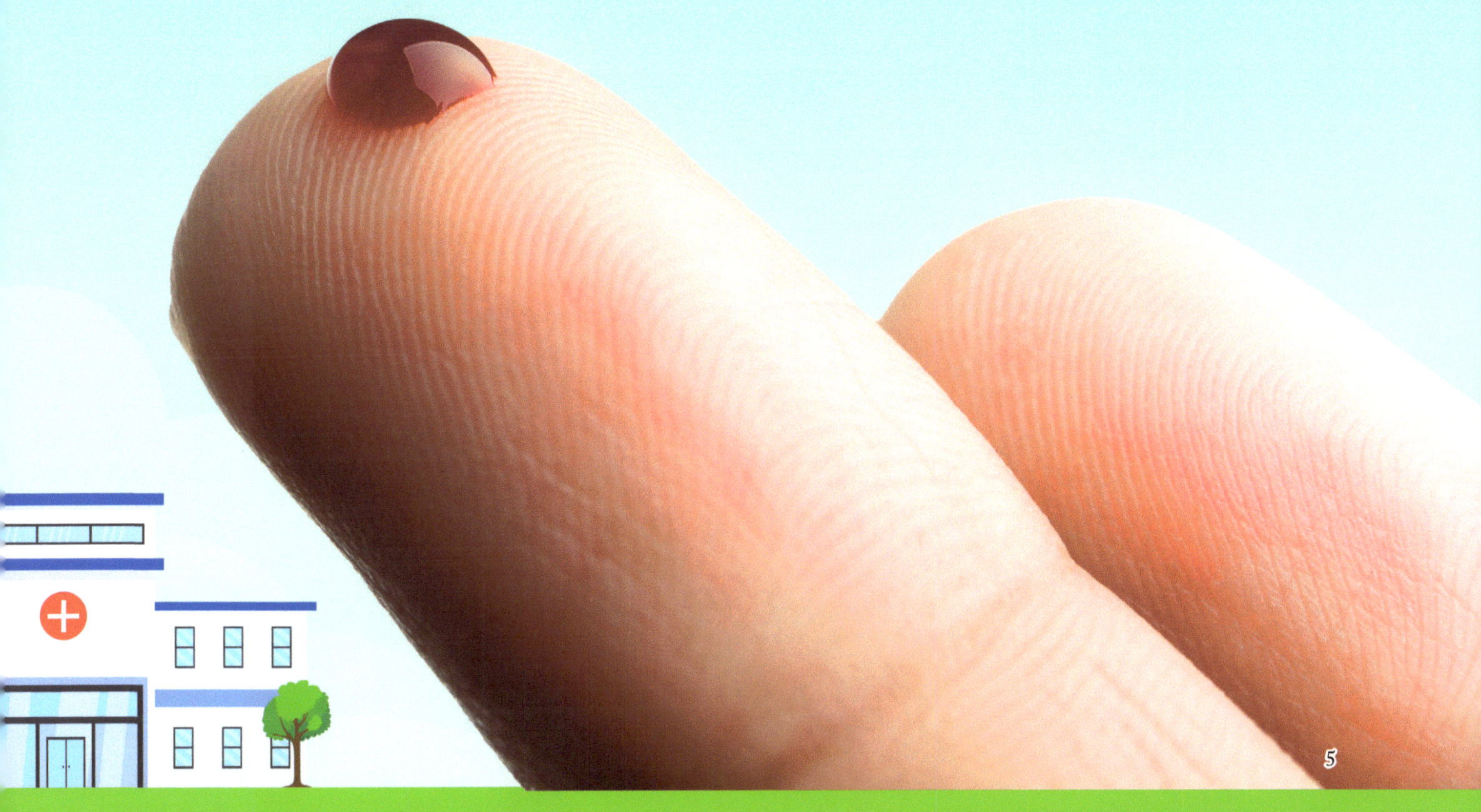

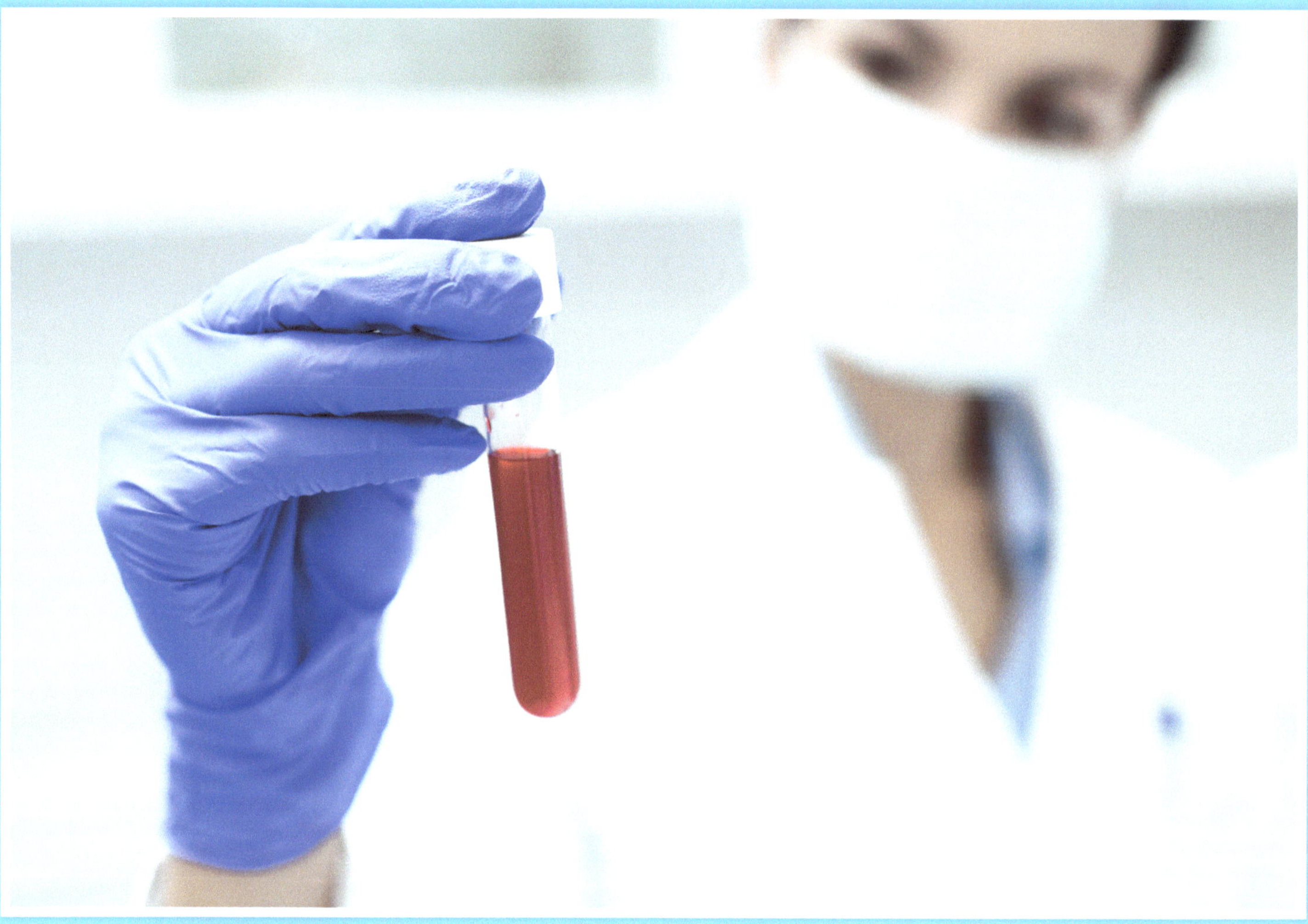

Sometimes a doctor needs to take out a little bit of your blood and test it to learn what's going on inside your body.

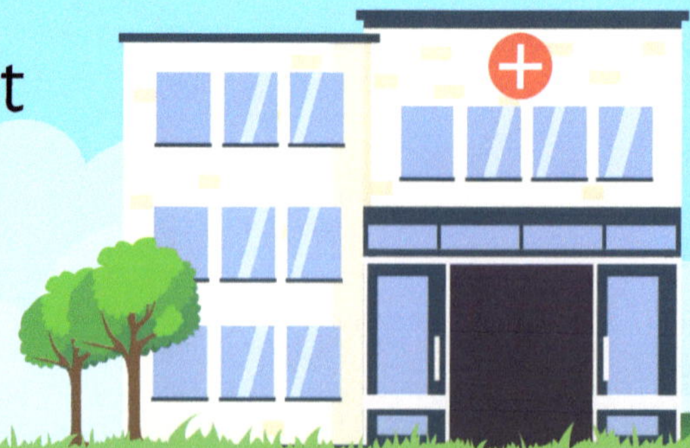

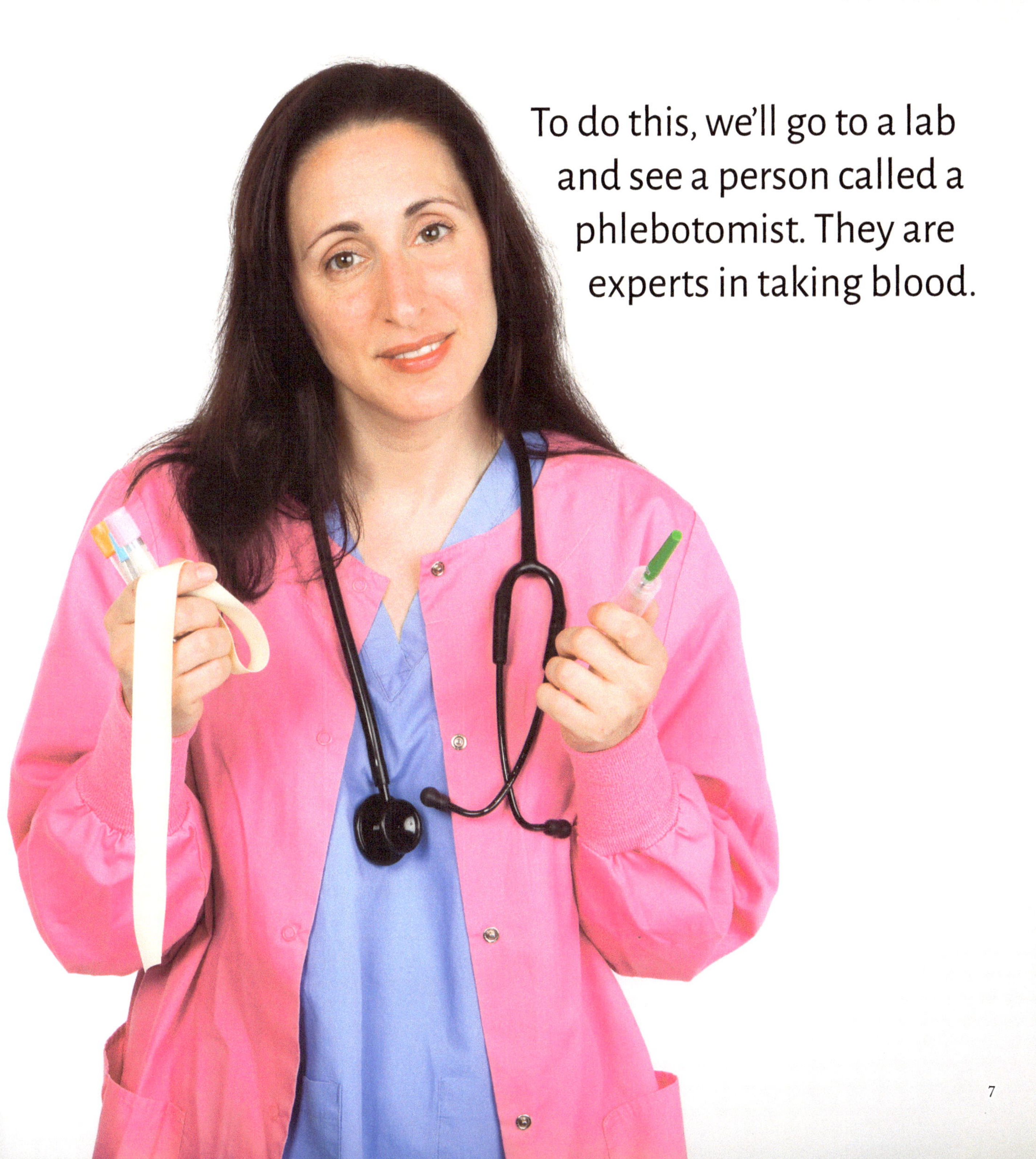

To do this, we'll go to a lab and see a person called a phlebotomist. They are experts in taking blood.

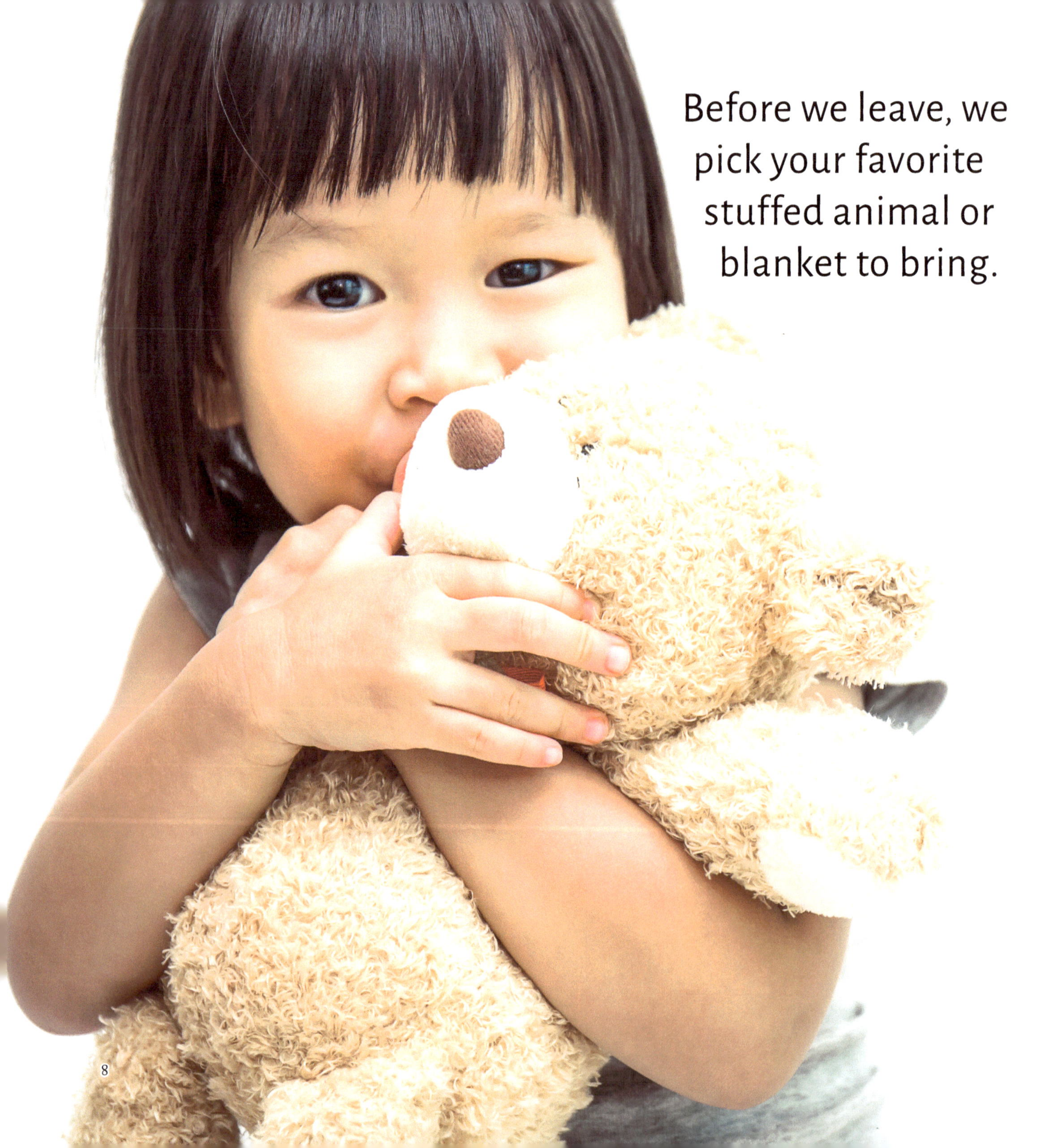

Before we leave, we pick your favorite stuffed animal or blanket to bring.

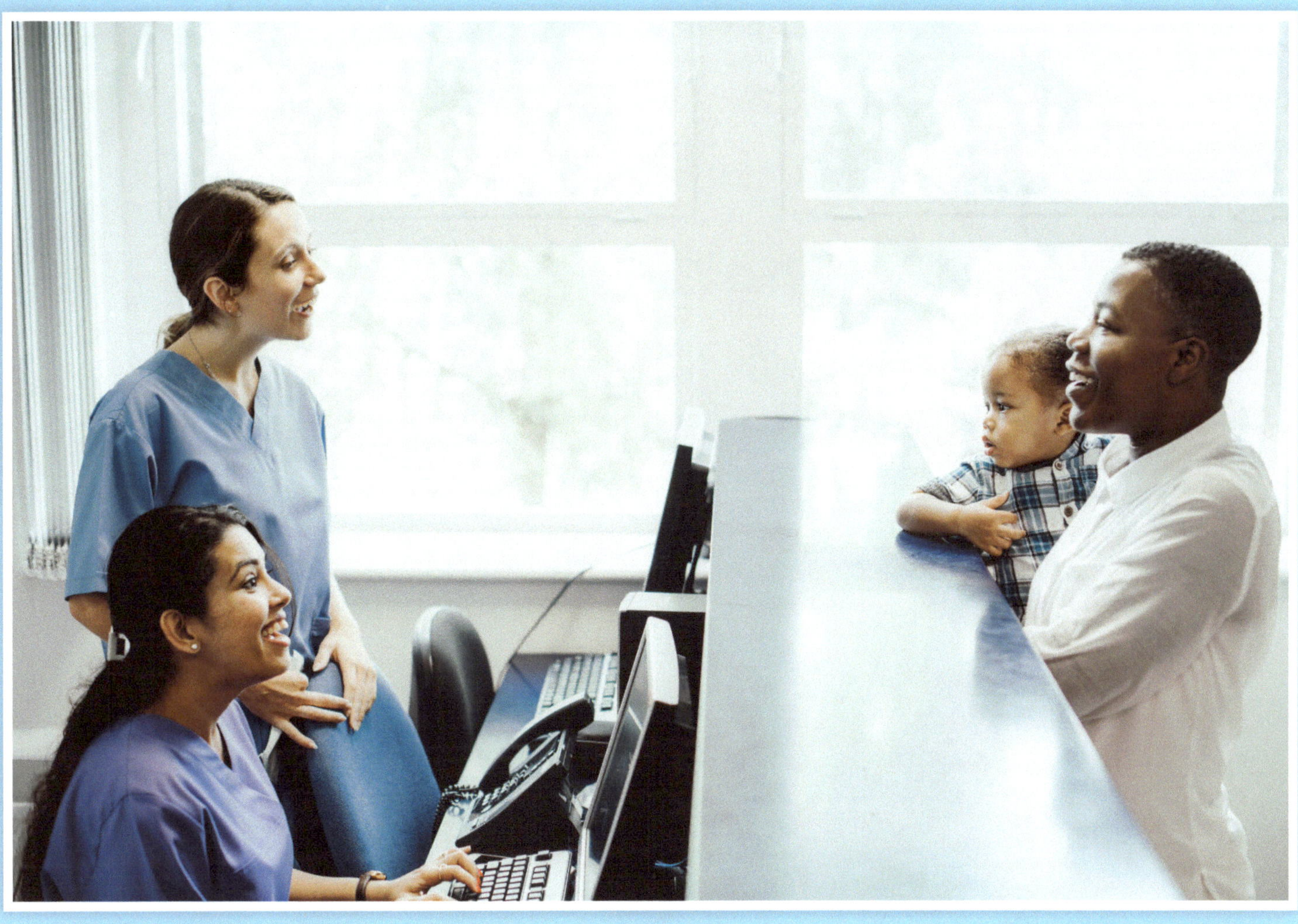

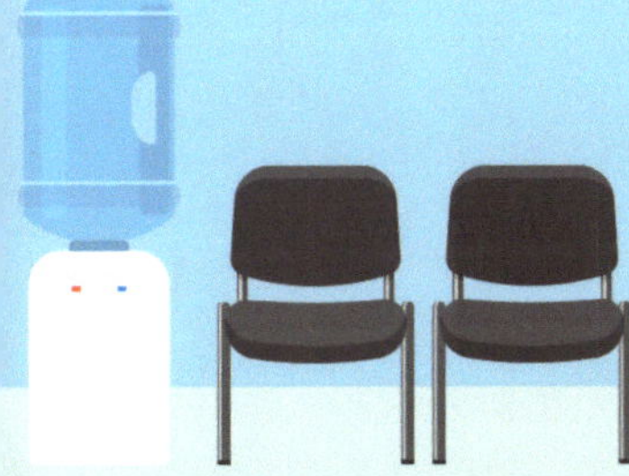

Then, we drive to the lab and check in at the front desk.

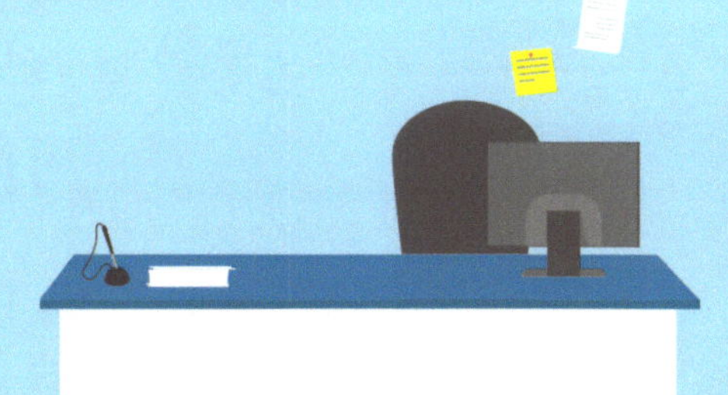

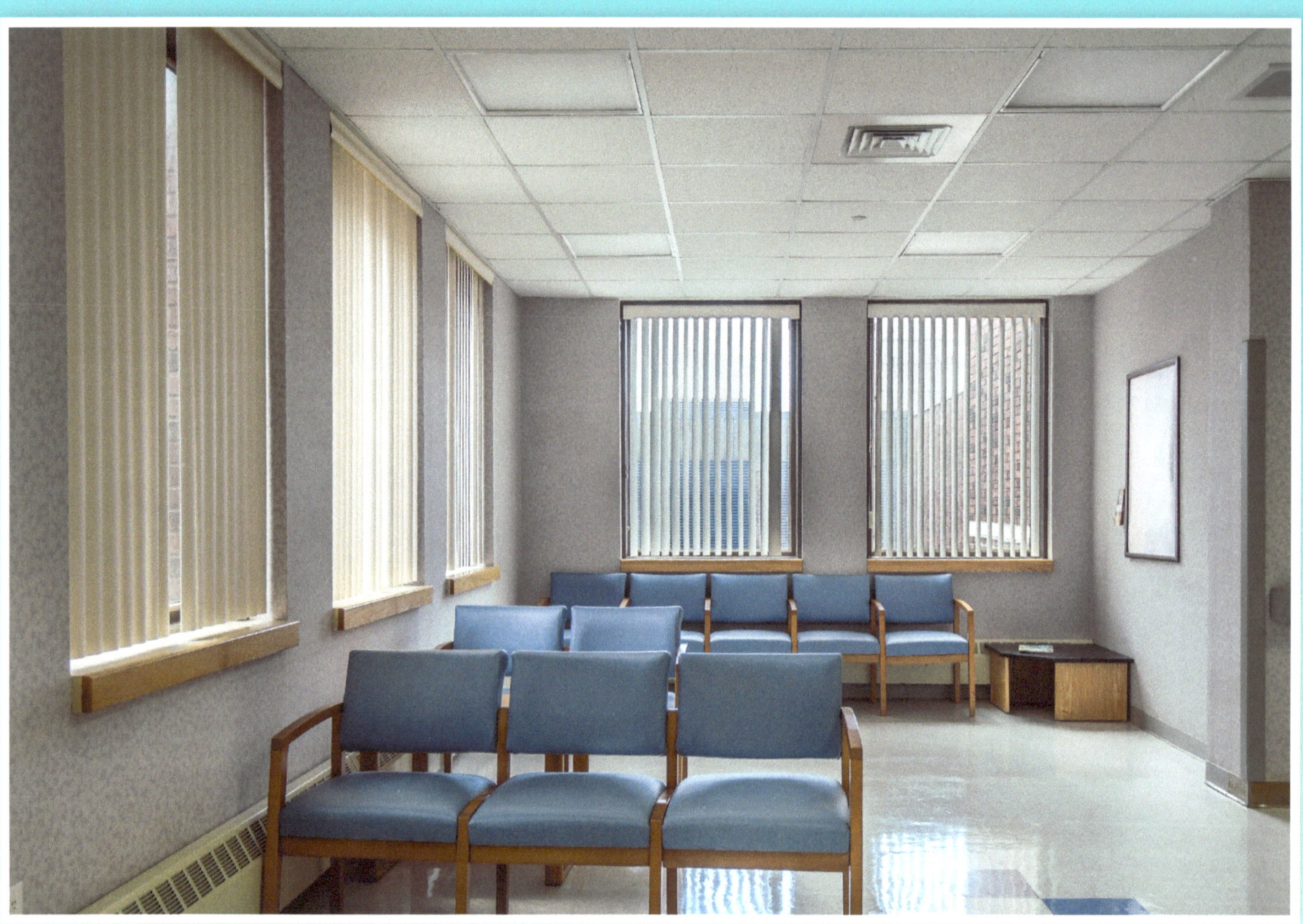

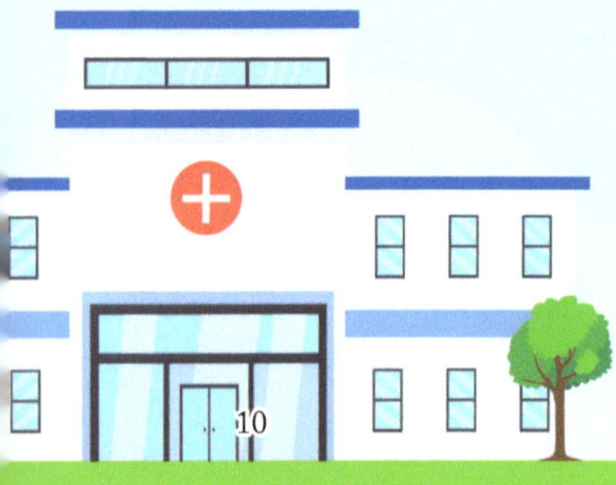

After we check in, we wait for your turn in the waiting room.

Then, the phlebotomist calls your name and takes us to a room.

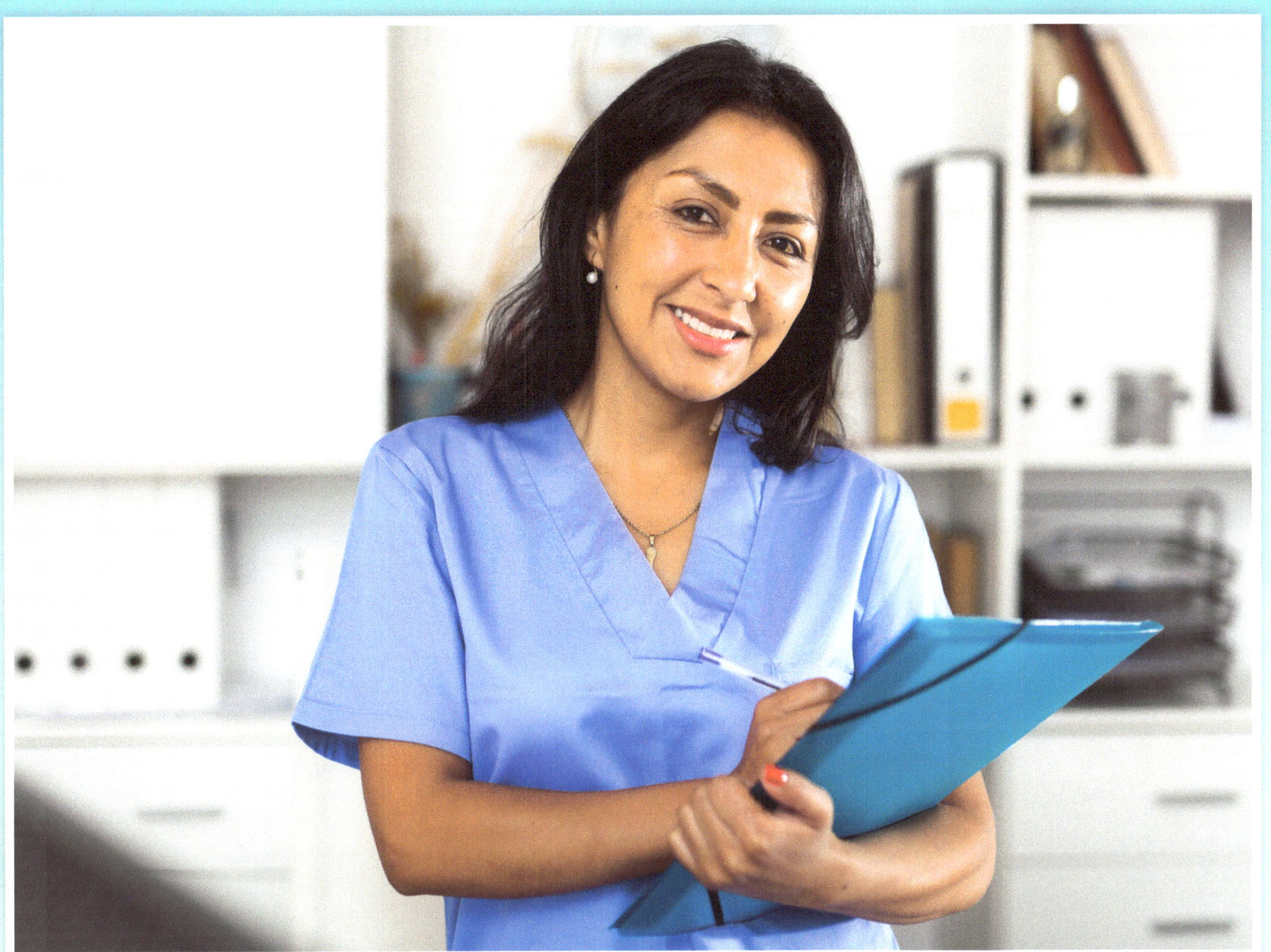

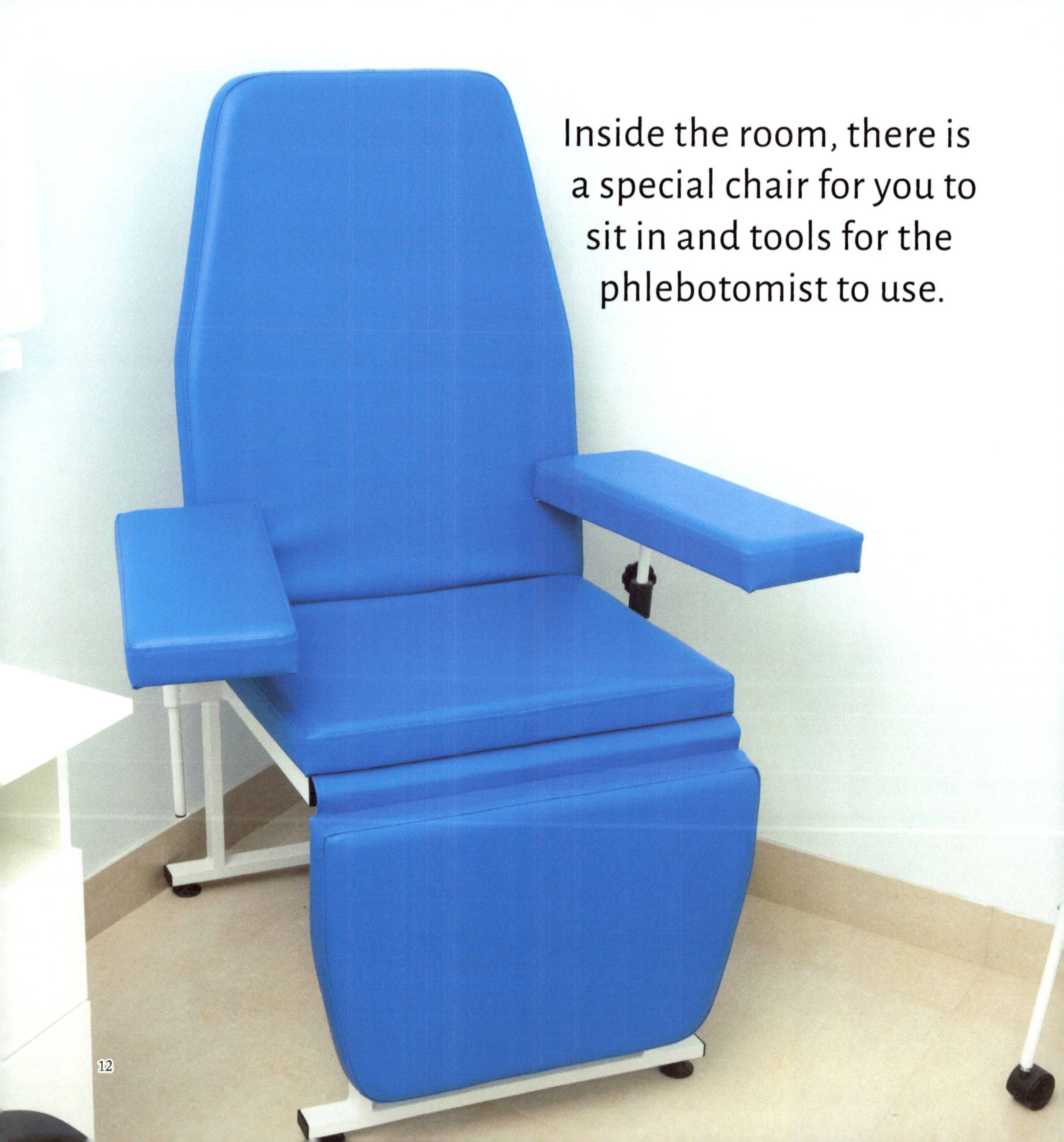
Inside the room, there is a special chair for you to sit in and tools for the phlebotomist to use.

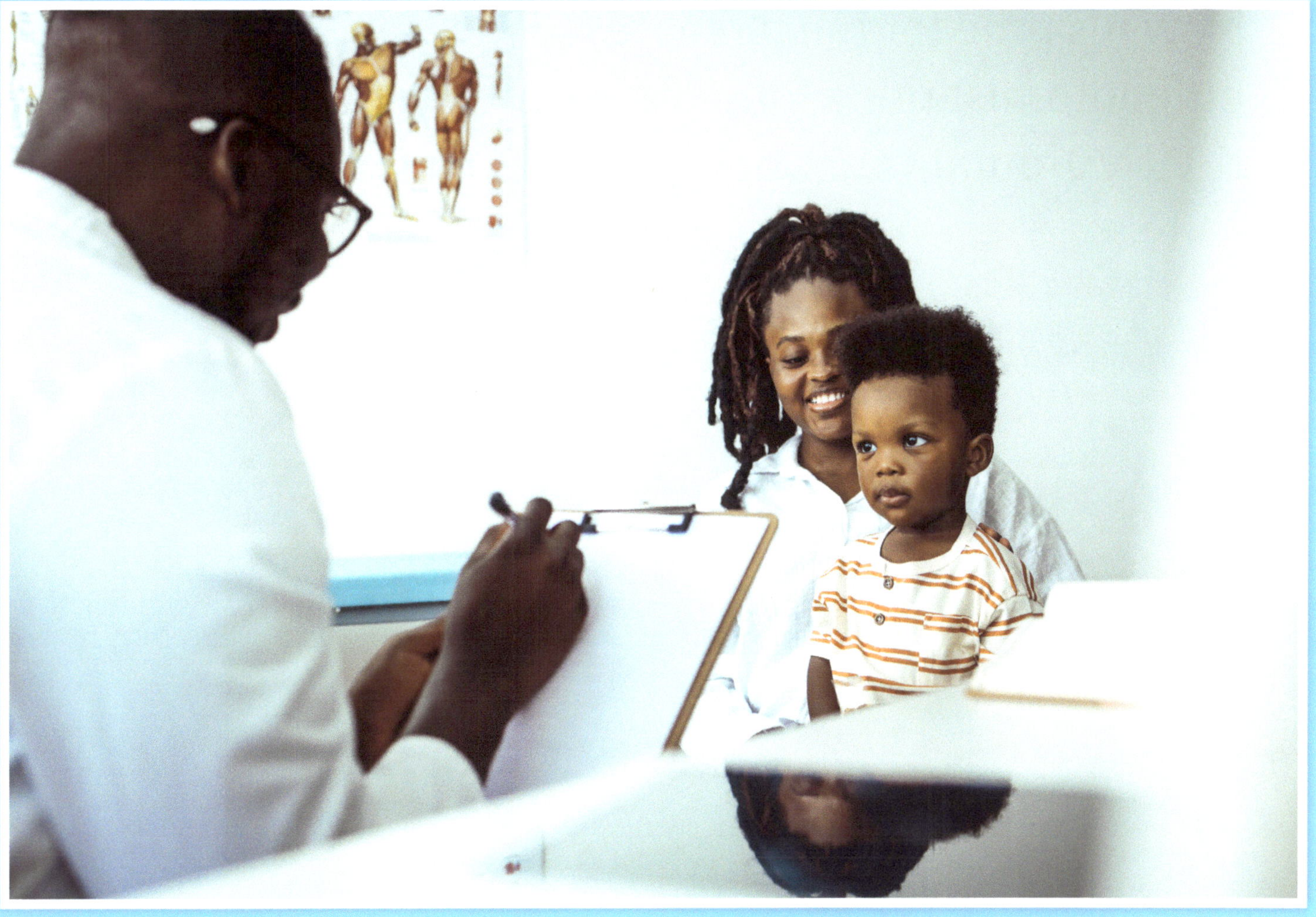

You can sit by yourself, or you can sit in my lap.

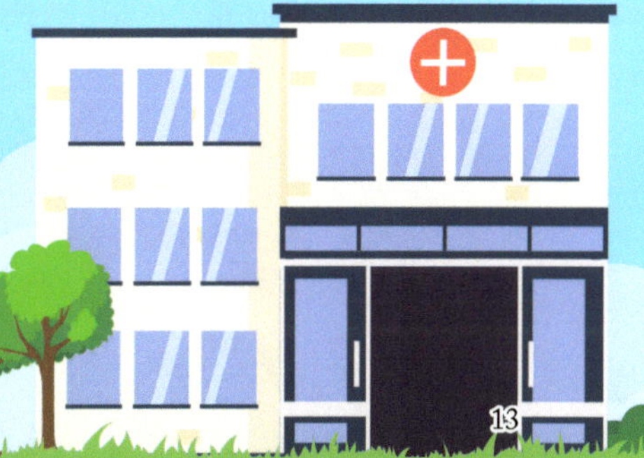

Now it's time for the blood test. First, the phlebotomist ties a long piece of rubber or fabric tightly around your arm.

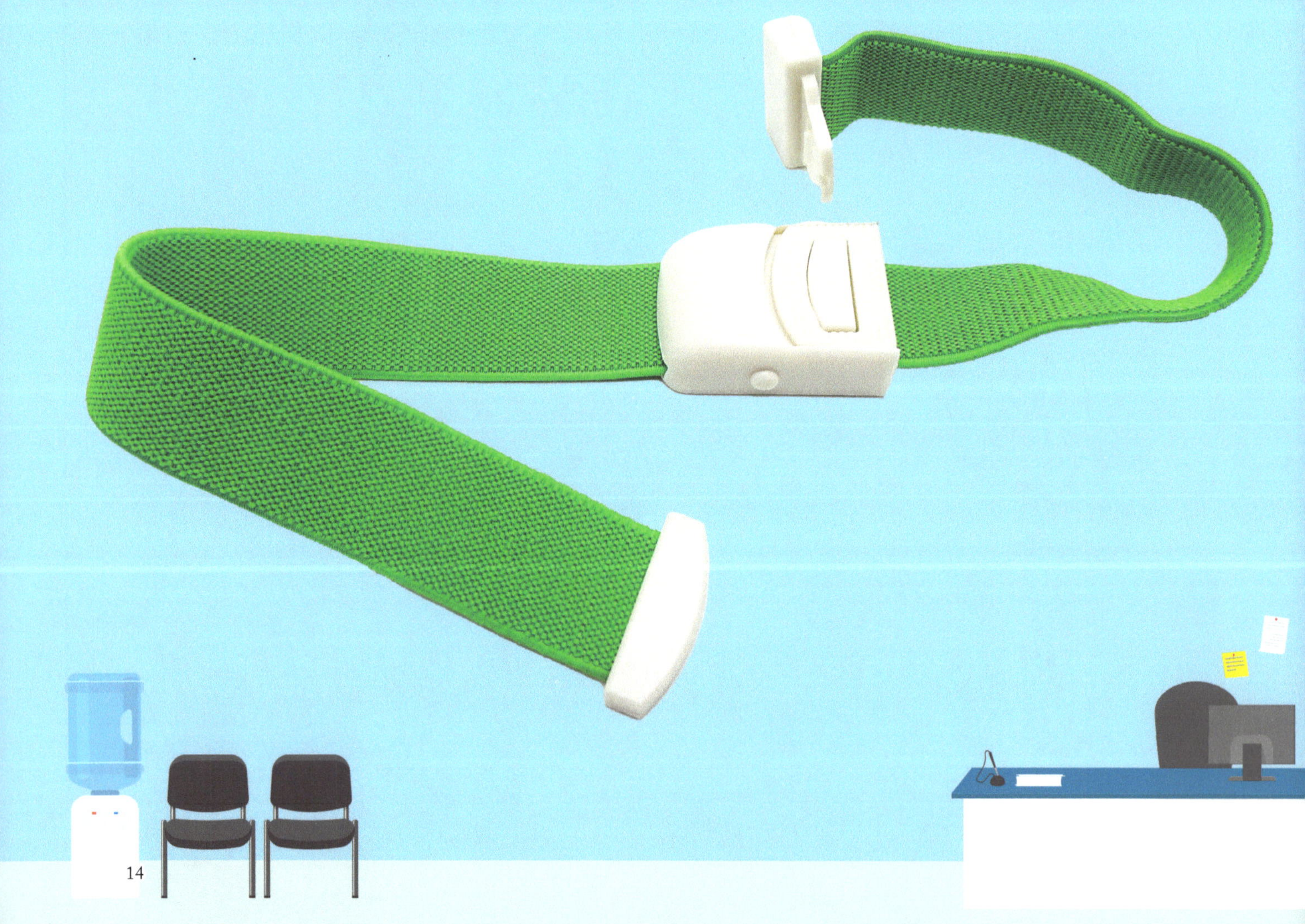

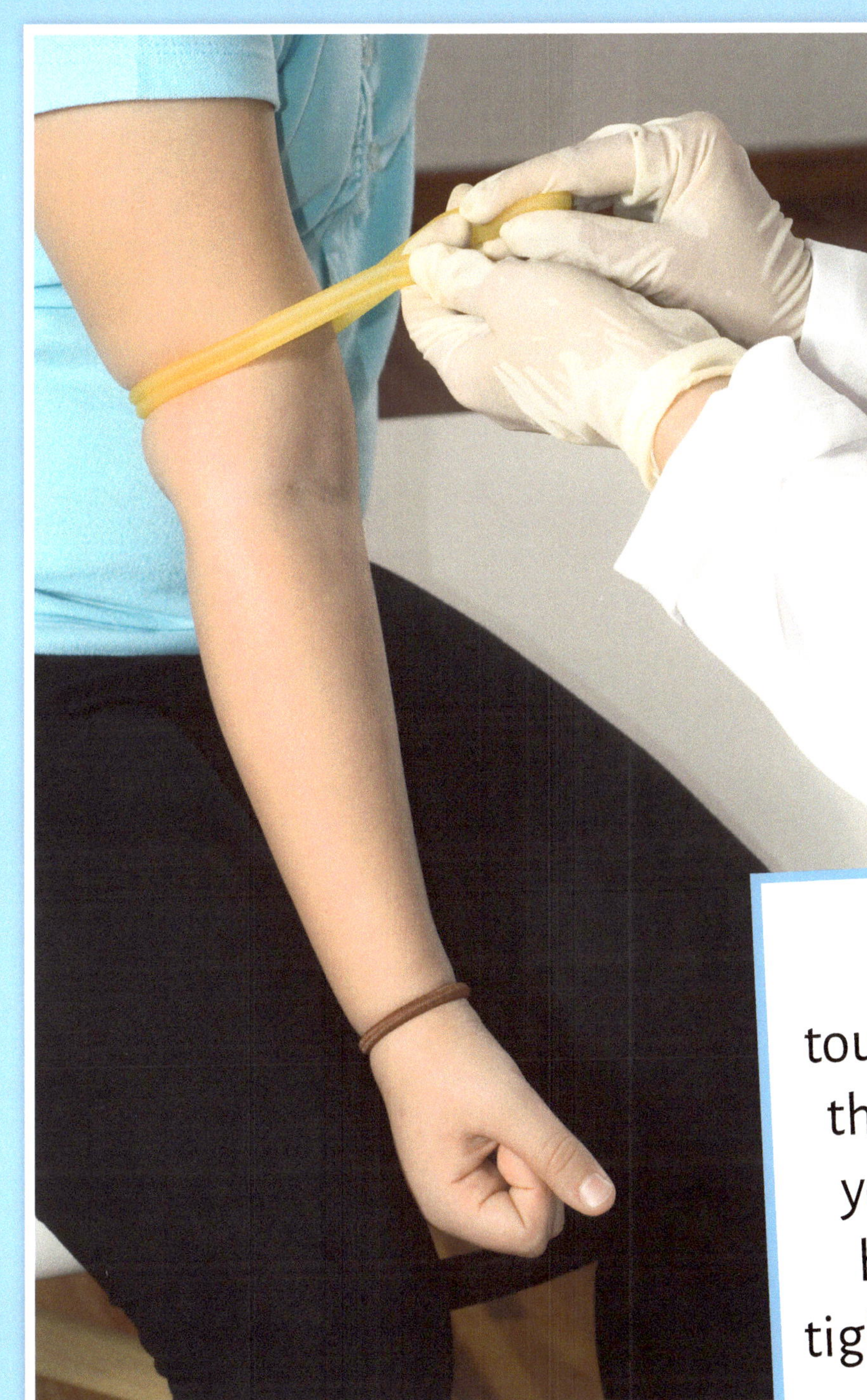

This is called a tourniquet and it helps the phlebotomist see your veins. It doesn't hurt, you just feel a tight squeeze like a hug.

Next, they clean your arm with a small wipe. It feels cold and smells a little funny.

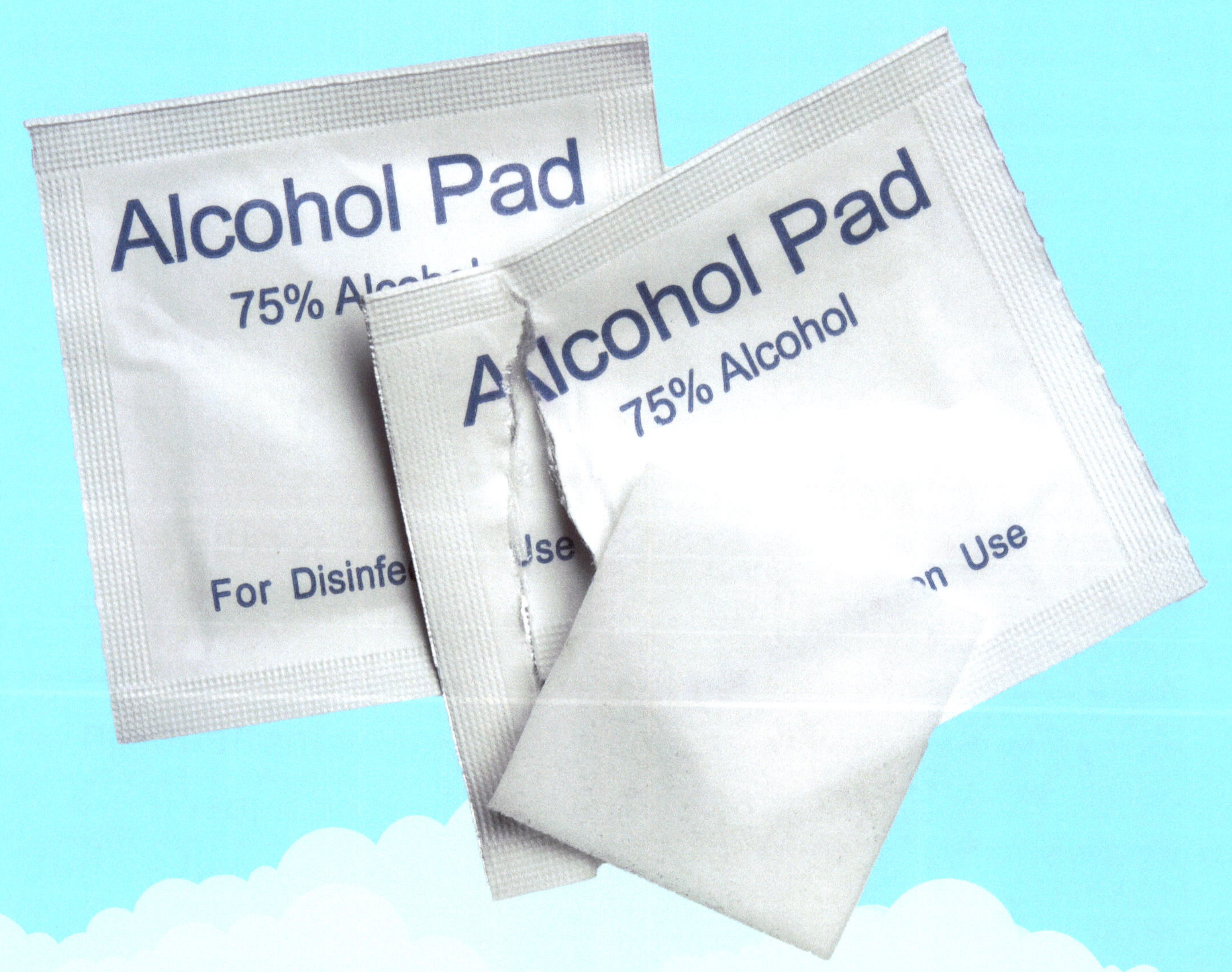

Then, the phlebotomist takes a very small needle and pokes your arm. Just like a shot, a blood test hurts a little, but not for long. It's important you hold very still.

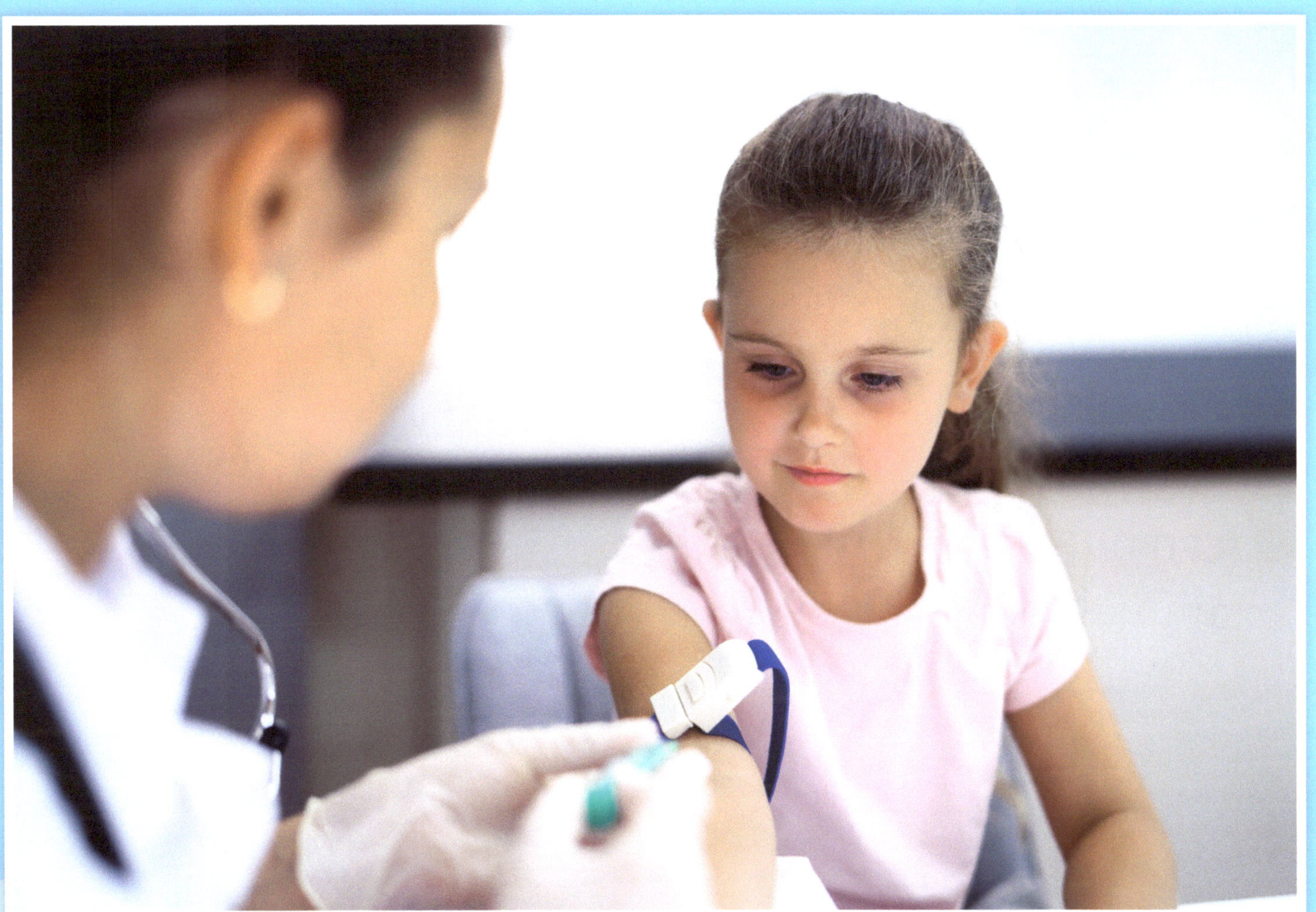

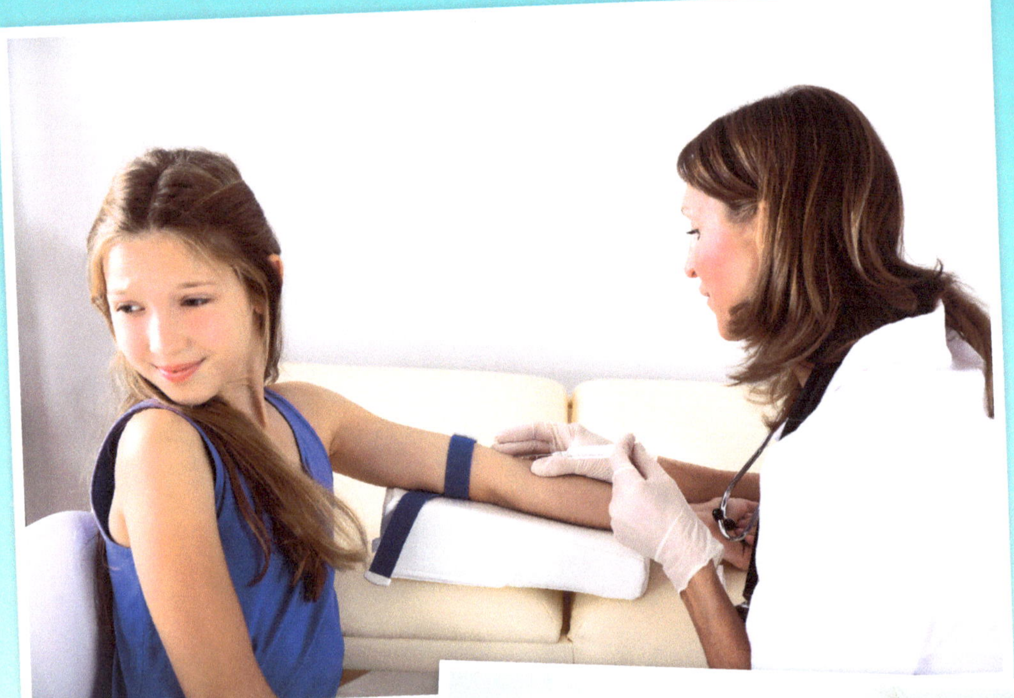

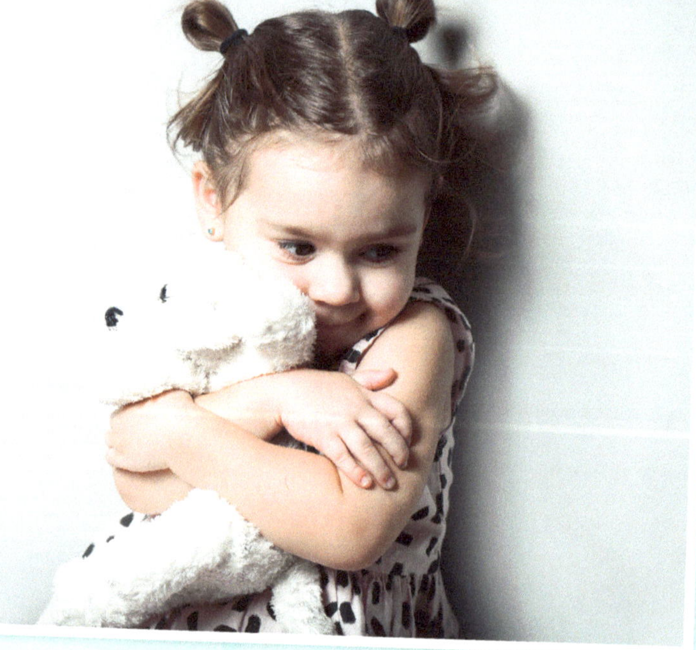

It's ok if you feel a little nervous. You can hug your stuffed animal or look at me.

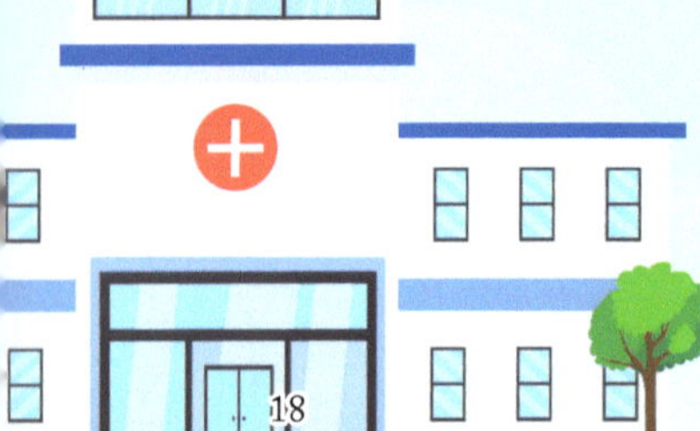

18

You continue to hold very still while the phlebotomist fills a couple viles of your blood. This doesn't take long.

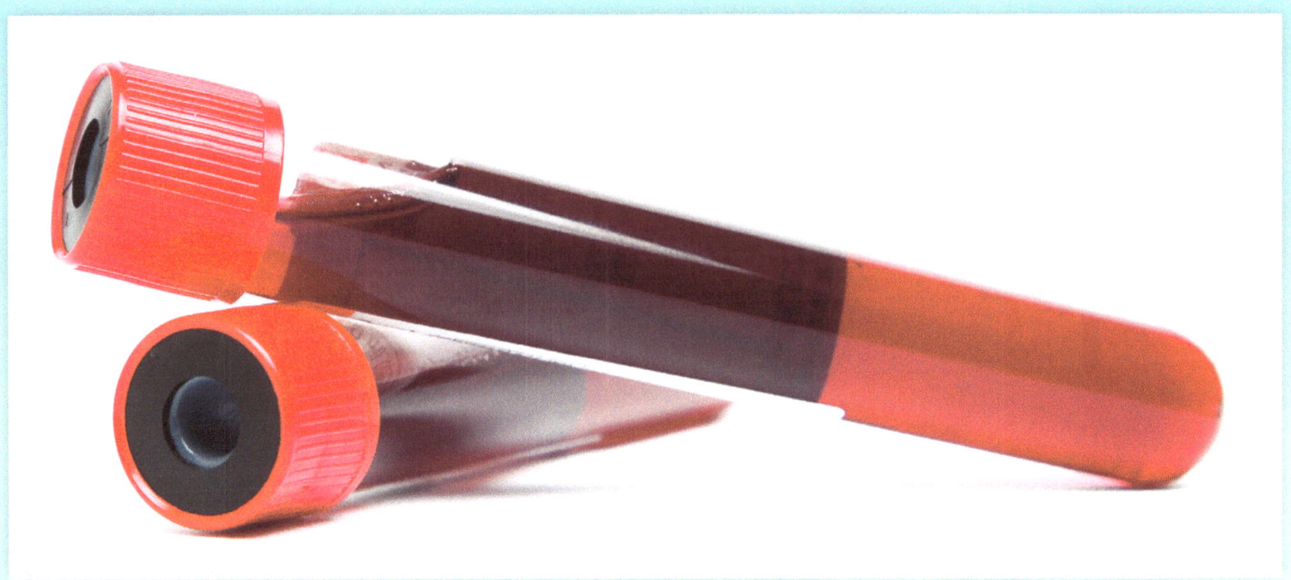

Finally, the phlebotomist puts a bandage on your arm and you're all done! Great job!

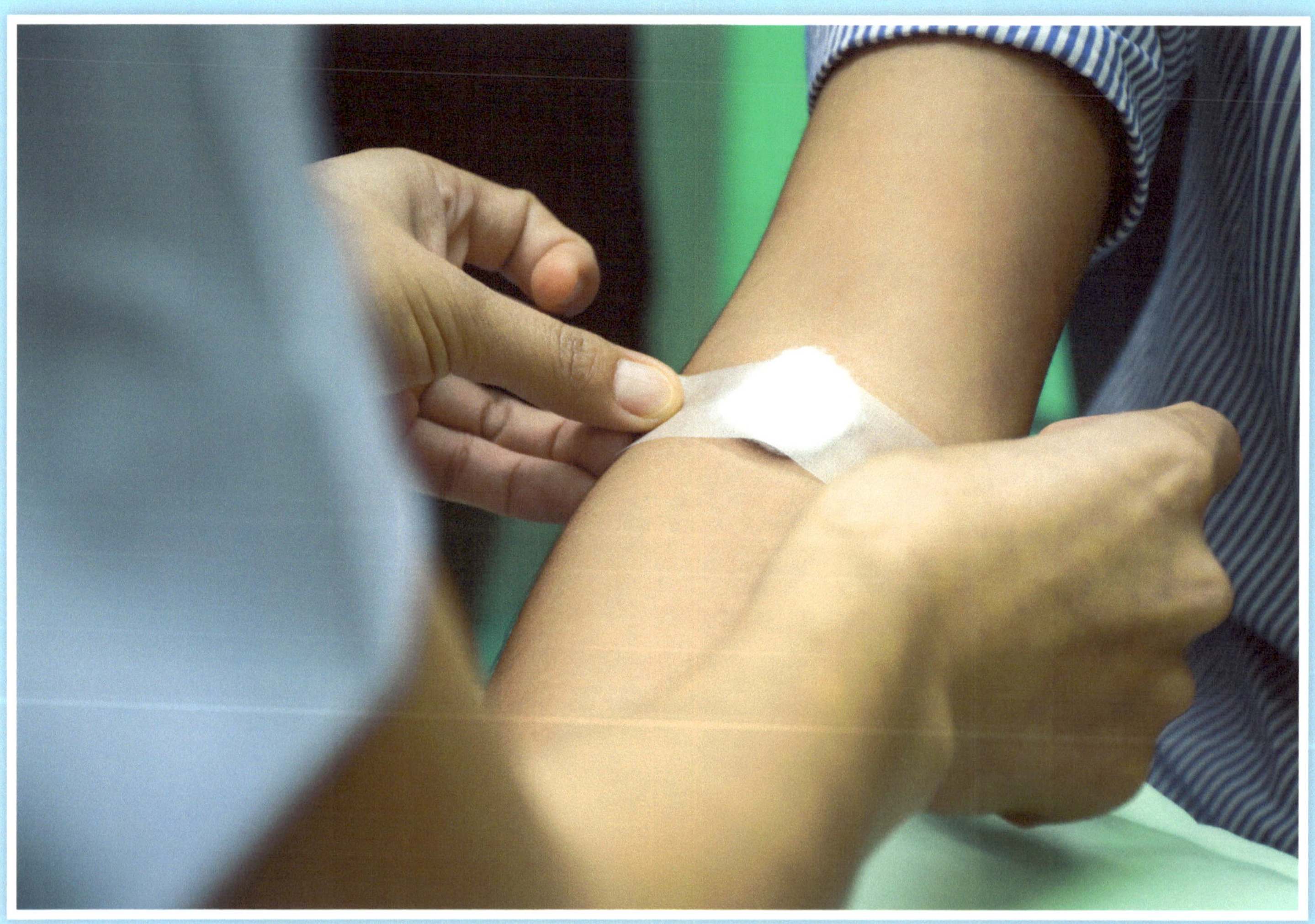

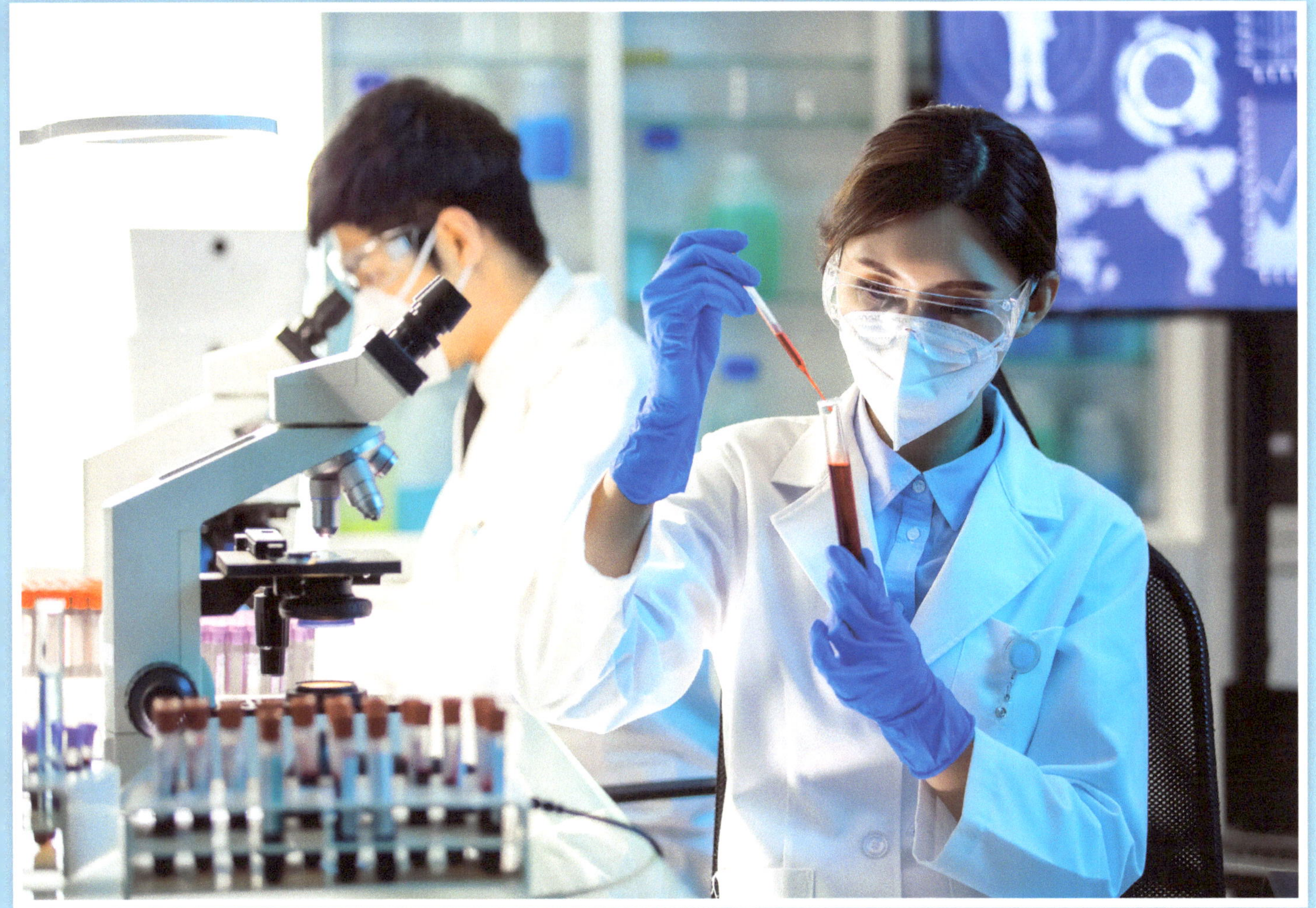

After we leave, the phlebotomist sends your blood away to the lab. They will look at it under a microscope to learn more about your body.

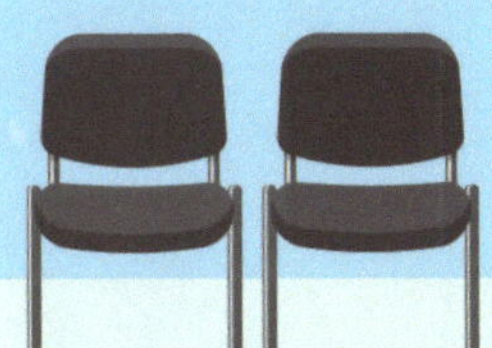

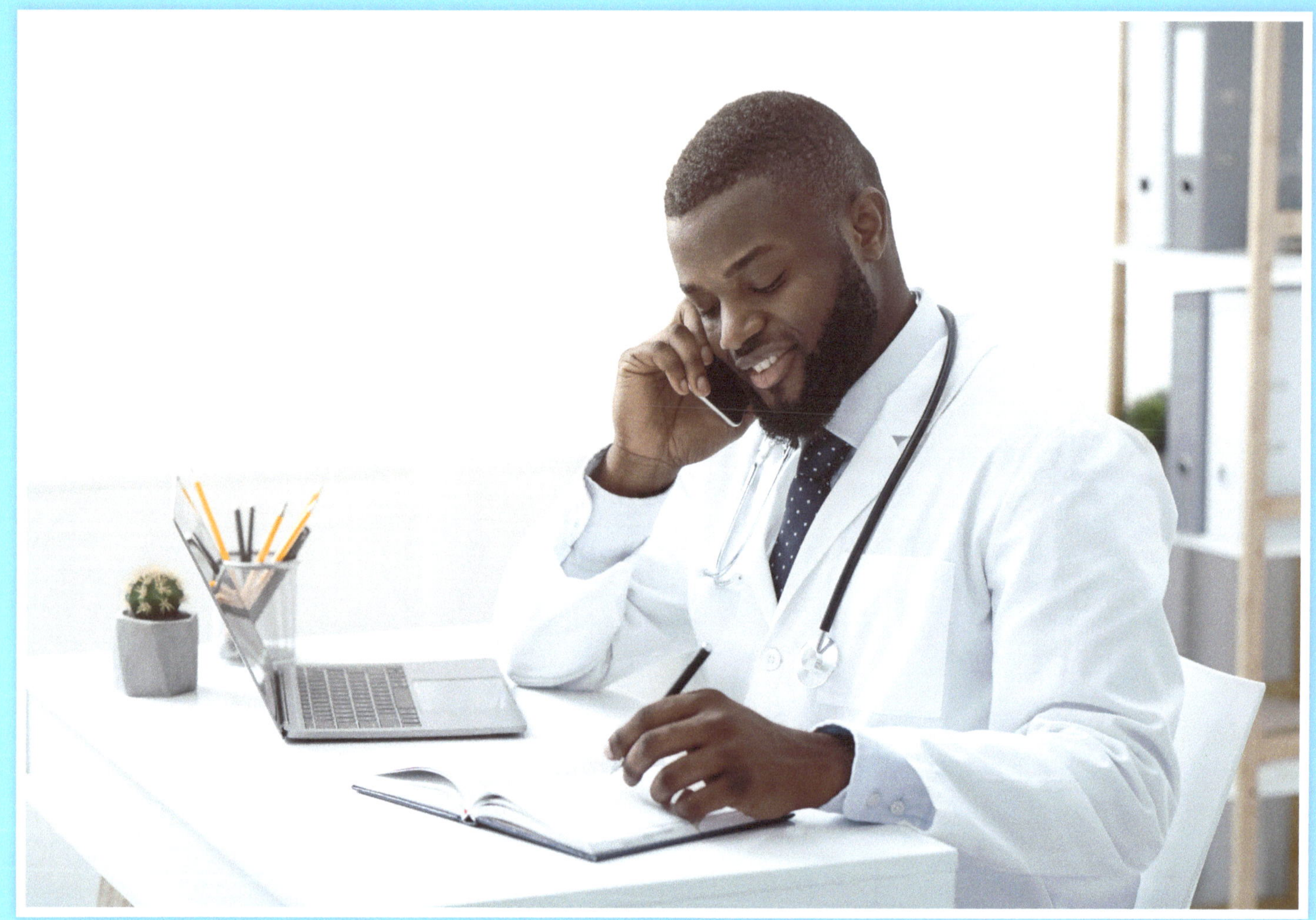

In a few weeks, the doctor calls us with the results of your blood test and we'll understand your body even better and how to keep it healthy.

Now you know all about getting a blood test.

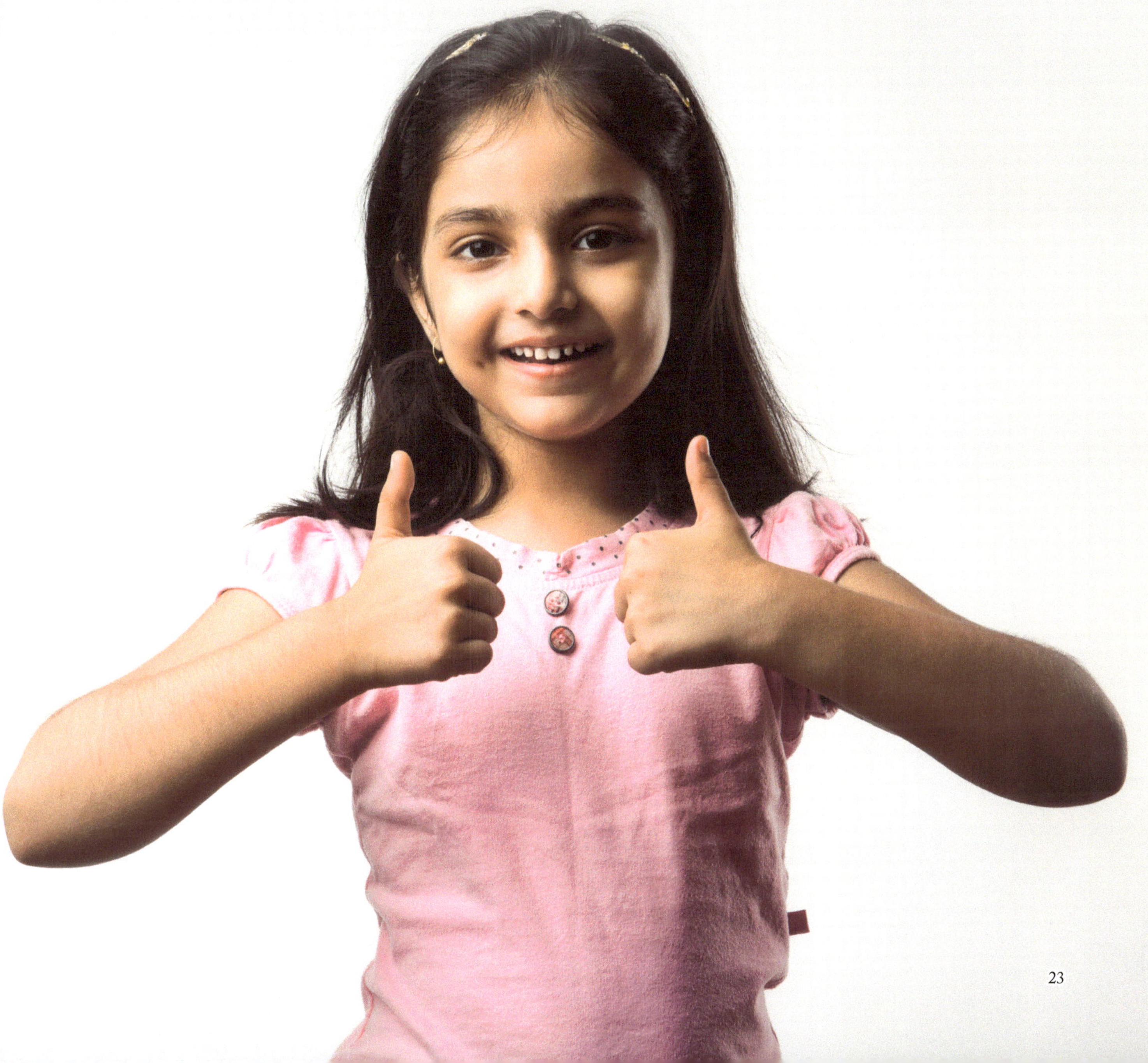